# RENAL ROADMAP:
# A Practical Guide To Understanding And Managing Kidney Disease.

## BY ASHLEY R. WHITLOW

# TABLE OF CONTENT

# INTRODUCTION TO THE KIDNEY

Your kidneys are responsible for removing waste and excess fluid from your body. Your kidneys also eliminate acid created by your body's cells and maintain a healthy balance of water, salts, and minerals in your blood, such as sodium, calcium, phosphorus, and potassium.

The kidneys are two bean-shaped organs that are around the size of a fist. They are placed on either side of your spine, directly below the rib cage. Every minute, healthy kidneys filter roughly a half cup of blood, eliminating wastes and excess water to produce urine. Urine travels from the kidneys to the bladder through two thin muscular tubes called ureters, one on each side of the bladder. Urine is stored in your bladder. The urinary tract includes your kidneys, ureters, and bladder.

# WHAT IS THE SIGNIFICANCE OF THE KIDNEYS?

Your kidneys are responsible for removing waste and excess fluid from your body. Your kidneys also eliminate acid created by your body's cells and maintain a healthy balance of water, salts, and minerals in your blood, such as sodium, calcium, phosphorus, and potassium.

Nerves, muscles, and other tissues in your body may not function correctly if this equilibrium is not maintained. Your kidneys also produce hormones that aid with digestion. keep your blood pressure under control. Each of your kidneys is composed of around a million filtering units known as nephrons. Each nephron has a filter called the glomerulus as well as a tubule.

***The nephrons filter your blood in two steps:*** the glomerulus filters it, and the tubule restores required chemicals to your blood while removing wastes. Your blood is filtered by the glomerulus. As blood rushes into each nephron, it enters the glomerulus, a network of microscopic blood arteries. The glomerulus' thin walls enable smaller molecules, wastes, and fluid—mostly water—to enter the tubule. Proteins and blood cells, for example, remain in the blood vessel. The tubule transports wastes and restores required chemicals to your blood. A blood artery runs parallel to the tubule. The blood vessel reabsorbs virtually all of the water, as well as minerals and nutrients, as the filtered fluid passes down the tubule. The tubule aids in the removal of excess acid from the circulation. Urine is formed from the leftover fluid and wastes in the tubule.

## WHAT IS THE FLOW OF BLOOD VIA MY KIDNEYS?

The renal artery allows blood to enter your kidney. This huge blood channel divides into smaller blood vessels until the blood reaches the nephrons. Your blood is filtered in the nephron by the microscopic blood vessels of the glomeruli before exiting your kidney through the renal vein. Your blood passes through your kidneys many times every day. Your kidneys filter around 150 quarts of blood every day. The tubules return the majority of the water and other chemicals that filter through your glomeruli to your blood. Only 1 to 2 quarts are converted to urine. Children generate less pee than adults, and the quantity they produce varies with age.

**WHAT EXACTLY IS KIDNEY DISEASE?**
Doctors use the phrase "kidney disease" to describe any abnormalities of the kidneys, even if the harm is minor. It is often referred to as 'chronic' renal disease. Chronic is a medical phrase that refers to a condition that does not improve entirely in a few days. A kidney condition, such as a simple urine infection that clears itself and leaves no harm, is not chronic kidney disease. According to recent studies, one in every ten people has mild renal disease. This is much more prevalent in the elderly than in the young.

In most situations, kidney disease is identified because tests are abnormal and do not produce any symptoms. These may include blood or protein tests in the urine, an X-ray or scan of the kidneys, or a blood test to assess kidney function. In many situations, the kidneys may continue to function for years without becoming very ill.

## WHAT IS KIDNEY FAILURE?

Kidney failure is a medical word that may be difficult to understand since it refers to decreased kidney function, which is generally less than 30% of normal (or estimated renal function of less than 30). Certain patients with kidney failure feel OK, and in certain situations, the kidneys may continue to function for years without deteriorating significantly.

## DOES EVERY KIDNEY DISEASE RESULT IN KIDNEY FAILURE?

The vast majority of patients with kidney disease have mild issues and never acquire renal failure. However, it is typical for patients with renal disease to have high blood pressure and circulatory difficulties, necessitating certain testing and continuing therapy. Overall, fewer than one in every ten people with renal disease will develop kidney failure.

## CAN I PREVENT KIDNEY FAILURE AFTER I HAVE KIDNEY DISEASE?

The long-term prognosis is determined by the kind of kidney disease present and the degree of the illness. These issues will need to be explored with the medical staff separately.

# CHAPTER 1: TYPES OF KIDNEY DISEASE

*Acute renal Disease* (CKD) and *Chronic Renal Disease* are the two primary kinds of kidney disease.

*Acute renal failure* happens when your kidneys abruptly stop filtering waste items from your blood. When your kidneys lose their filtering abilities, harmful quantities of waste may collect, and the chemical composition of your blood can go out of balance.

## ACUTE RENAL DISEASE

Acute kidney failure, also known as acute renal failure or acute kidney damage, occurs quickly, generally within a few days. Acute renal failure is more likely in those who are already hospitalized, especially those who are seriously sick and need intensive care. Acute renal failure may be deadly and need immediate medical attention. Acute renal failure, on the other hand, may be reversible. If you are generally healthy, you may be able to regain normal or almost normal kidney function.

**SYMPTOMS OF ACUTE RENAL DISEASE**

1. Urine production is reduced, while it sometimes stays normal.

2. Swelling in your legs, ankles, or feet due to fluid retention Breathing difficulty.

3. Fatigue.

4. Nausea.

5. Weakness Heartbeat irregularity Pain, or pressure in the chest In extreme circumstances, seizures or coma may occur.

Sometimes acute renal failure has no symptoms and is discovered via blood testing performed for another reason. If you experience signs or symptoms of acute renal failure, consult your doctor right away or seek emergency treatment. If your signs and symptoms point to acute renal failure, your doctor may advise you to undergo specific tests and treatments to confirm your diagnosis.

**ACUTE KIDNEY DISEASE TEST**

*1. Measuring urine production.* Measuring how much you urinate in 24 hours might help your doctor figure out what's causing your kidney failure. Urine tests are performed.

*2. A urine test (urinalysis).* This may detect abnormalities that indicate renal failure. Blood tests are performed. A blood sample may indicate rapidly increasing levels of urea and creatinine, two chemicals used to assess kidney function.

*3. Imaging examinations.* Ultrasound and computed tomography imaging tests may be done to assist your doctor visualize your kidneys.

*4. Taking a kidney tissue sample for examination.* In certain cases, your doctor may advise you to have a kidney biopsy to get a tiny sample of kidney tissue for laboratory testing. To extract the sample, the doctor inserts a needle through your skin and into your kidney. When most patients suffer acute renal failure, they are already in the hospital. Bring your worries to your doctor or nurse if you or a loved one develops signs and symptoms of renal failure. If you are not in the hospital but are experiencing signs or symptoms of renal failure, see your family doctor or a general practitioner. If your doctor believes you have kidney disease, you may be sent to a nephrologist (a doctor who specializes in renal illness).

Make a list of your questions before visiting with the doctor. Consider the following:
*What may be the most likely source of my symptoms?
*Have my kidneys ceased functioning?
*What may have been the reason for my renal failure?
*What kind of exams do I require?
* What are my treatment choices, and what are the dangers associated with them?
*Is it necessary for me to go to the hospital?
*Will my kidneys heal or will I need dialysis?
*Do I need to follow a specific diet, and if so,

can you recommend a dietician to assist me plan my meals?

## TREATMENT

A hospital stay is usually required for the treatment of acute renal failure. The majority of persons with acute renal failure are already in the hospital. The length of your hospital stay is determined by the cause of your acute renal failure and how fast your kidneys recover. You may be able to heal at home in certain circumstances. Identifying the infection or injury that caused your kidneys to fail is the first step in treating acute renal failure. Your treatment choices are determined by the cause of your renal failure.

## COMPLICATION-PREVENTION TREATMENTS

Treatments to balance the fluid levels in your blood. Your doctor may offer intravenous (IV) fluids if your acute kidney failure is caused by a shortage of fluids in your blood. In some circumstances, severe renal failure may cause you to retain too much fluid, resulting in arm and leg edema. In certain circumstances, your doctor may prescribe diuretics, which cause your body to remove excess fluids. Medications that regulate blood potassium levels. If your kidneys aren't filtering potassium from your blood adequately, your doctor may give calcium, glucose, or sodium polystyrene sulfonate (Kionex) to avoid excessive potassium levels in your blood.

A high potassium level in the bloodstream may lead to serious irregular heartbeats (arrhythmias) and muscular weakness. Medications that increase blood calcium levels. If the calcium levels in your blood become too low, your doctor may consider a calcium infusion. Dialysis is used to eliminate toxins from the blood. If toxins accumulate in your blood, you may need temporary hemodialysis, also known as dialysis, to help eliminate toxins and extra fluids from your body while your kidneys repair.

Dialysis may also aid in the removal of excess potassium from your body. A machine pumps blood out of your body via an artificial kidney (dialyzer) that filters out waste during dialysis. After that, the blood is returned to your body.

## DIET TIPS DURING YOUR RECOVERY FROM ACUTE RENAL FAILURE

your doctor may advise you to follow a particular diet to assist your kidneys and reduce the amount of work they have to perform.
Your doctor may send you to a dietician who may assess your current diet and provide recommendations to make it easier on your kidneys.

Depending on your circumstances, your dietician may advise you to:
1. Choose foods that are low in potassium.
Bananas, oranges, potatoes, spinach, and tomatoes are high in potassium. Apples, cauliflower, peppers, grapes, and strawberries are examples of low-potassium foods.

2. Reduce your daily sodium intake by avoiding foods with excess salt, which includes many convenience meals such as frozen dinners, canned soups, and fast foods. Other salty snack items, canned veggies, processed meats, and cheeses include additional salt.

3. Phosphorus should be kept to a minimum. Phosphorus is a mineral that may be found in whole-grain bread, oats, bran cereals, dark-colored colas, almonds, and peanut butter. Too much phosphorous in your blood may cause bone weakness and skin irritation. Your dietician may provide you with precise phosphorus guidelines. As your kidneys heal, you may no longer need a particular diet, while good eating is always necessary.

**CHRONIC KIDNEY DISEASE**

Chronic kidney disease, commonly known as ***chronic kidney failure,*** is characterized by a progressive decrease in renal function. Wastes and surplus fluids in your blood are filtered by your kidneys and excreted in your urine.

Advanced chronic renal disease may result in dangerously high amounts of fluid, electrolytes, and wastes in your body. You may have minimal indications or symptoms in the early stages of chronic renal disease. You may not notice you have renal disease until it is too late.

Chronic renal disease treatment focuses on delaying the course of kidney damage, generally by addressing the underlying cause. However, even if the cause is not controlled, kidney damage may worsen. Chronic kidney disease may lead to end-stage renal failure, which is deadly without dialysis or a kidney transplant.

**CAUSES OF CHRONIC KIDNEY DISEASE**
Chronic kidney disease occurs when a disease or condition compromises kidney function, causing kidney damage to worsen over time. It is caused by a variety of diseases and situations, including;
1. Diabetes type 1 or diabetes type 2.
2. Blood pressure that is too high.
3. Glomerulonephritis: is an inflammation of the filtration units (glomeruli) of the kidney.

4. Interstitial nephritis is an inflammation of the tubules and surrounding tissues of the kidney.

5. Recurrent kidney infection pyelonephritis.

6. malignancies Vesicoureteral Reflux is a disorder in which pee backs up into your kidneys.

7. Other hereditary kidney illnesses such as polycystic kidney disease and Prolonged urinary tract blockage caused by disorders such as an enlarged prostate, kidney stones.

## SYMPTOMS OF CHRONIC KIDNEY DISEASE

If kidney damage proceeds slowly, signs and symptoms of chronic kidney disease emerge over time. Kidney failure may result in an accumulation of fluid or waste, as well as electrolyte imbalances. Depending on the severity, kidney function loss might result in: Nausea, Vomiting Appetite loss, fatigue, Sleep issues, urinating more or less often, Reduced mental acuity, Cramps in the muscles, Foot and ankle swelling, Itchy, dry skin, Hypertension (high blood pressure) that are difficult to manage

Shortness of breath if fluid accumulates in the lungs If fluid accumulates around the heart's lining, it may cause chest discomfort.

*The signs and symptoms of renal illness are often vague. This implies that they may be caused by other ailments as well. Because your kidneys can compensate for reduced function, you may not notice any symptoms until permanent damage has occurred.*

## When Should You Visit A Doctor?

If you have signs or symptoms of renal illness, make an appointment with your doctor. Early identification may aid in the prevention of renal disease developing into kidney failure. If you have a medical condition that raises your risk of kidney disease, your doctor may use urine and blood tests during office visits to check your blood pressure and kidney function. Consult your doctor to see whether these tests are essential for you.

**CAUSES OF CHRONIC KIDNEY DISEASE**

The following factors may raise your risk of chronic kidney disease:

1. Diabetes,

2. Blood pressure that is too high.

3. Cardiovascular (heart) disease.

4. Smoking.

5. Obesity.

6. Kidney structural abnormality.

7. Older age.

8. Use of drugs that may harm the kidneys regularly.

## COMPLICATIONS CHRONIC KIDNEY DISEASE

Complications Chronic kidney disease may impact almost every organ in the body.

Among the possible problems are:

1. ***Fluid retention:*** Fluid retention may cause arm and leg swelling, elevated blood pressure, and fluid in the lungs (pulmonary edema).

2. ***Increase in potassium levels:*** An abrupt increase in potassium levels in your blood (hyperkalemia), may damage heart function and be fatal.

3. Anemia, Cardiovascular disease ,Weak bones, and a higher risk of fractures Reduced sexual desire, erectile problems, or infertility Damage to your central nervous system . It might result in trouble focusing, personality problems, or seizures.
Reduced immunological response, making you more susceptible to infection

4. ***Pericarditis:*** This is an infection of the saclike membrane that surrounds and protects your heart (pericardium).

***Complications of pregnancy:*** It pose dangers to both the mother and the growing baby. The end-stage renal disease causes irreversible. kidney deterioration, necessitating dialysis or a kidney transplant for survival.

**PREVENTION**

To lower your chances of acquiring kidney disease do the following:

1. Take over-the-counter drugs exactly as directed.

2. Follow the directions on the box while using nonprescription pain medicines such as aspirin, ibuprofen (Advil, Motrin IB, and others), and acetaminophen (Tylenol, and others).

3. Taking too many pain medicines over an extended time may cause renal damage.

4. Keep a healthy weight. Maintain your healthy weight by being physically active most days of the week.

If you need to reduce weight, see your doctor about appropriate weight loss options.

5. You should not smoke. Cigarette smoking may harm your kidneys and aggravate pre-existing renal problems. If you smoke, speak to your doctor about quitting methods. Support groups, therapy, and drugs may all assist you in quitting. Manage your medical issues with the assistance of your doctor. Work with your doctor

to manage any illnesses or conditions that raise your risk of renal disease. Inquire with your doctor about tests to look for signs of kidney damage.

# CHAPTER 2: STAGES OF KIDNEY DISEASE

Chronic kidney disease is divided into five phases, beginning with a minimally damaged kidney and progressing to kidney failure. Treatments such as medicines and dialysis may keep your kidney disease from developing to stage 5.

Kidneys perform several functions that are critical to optimum health. They operate as blood filters, eliminating waste, poisons, and excess fluids. They also aid in maintaining bone health and increase red blood cell formation by regulating blood pressure and blood chemistry If you have chronic kidney disease (CKD), your kidneys have been damaged for more than a few months. Damaged kidneys can not filter blood as efficiently as they should, which may result in many major health issues. There are five phases of CKD, each with its own set of symptoms and therapies. The Centers for Disease Control and Prevention (CDC) estimates that 37 million individuals in the United States have CKD, yet the vast majority have not been diagnosed. It is a progressive disease, although therapy may reduce its progression. Not everyone develops renal failure.

A summary of the phases To assign a CKD stage, your doctor must first assess how effectively your kidneys function. A urine test to determine your albumin-creatinine ratio (ACR) is one method. It determines if the protein is seeping into the urine (proteinuria), a symptom of kidney disease. The following are the ACR levels: A1 less than 3mg/mmol, indicating a normal to modest rise A2 3-30mg/mmol, a little rise A3 more than 30mg/mmol, a significant rise.

To check the anatomy of your kidneys, your doctor may also request imaging tests such as an ultrasound. A blood test determines how effectively the kidneys perform by measuring creatinine, urea, and other waste products in the blood. A GFR of 100 mL/min is considered normal.

## THE FIVE PHASES OF CKD

The glomerular filtration rate, or GFR, measures how much blood your kidneys filter in one minute. GFR is calculated using a formula that takes into account body size, age, gender, and ethnicity. A GFR is as low as 60 might be deemed normal if there is no other sign of renal issues. GFR measures may be deceptive if you are a bodybuilder or have an eating disorder, for example. Kidney disease in its early stages

## STAGE 1

Kidney that is normal to highly functioning >90 mL/min >90%.

They're highly adaptive and can compensate for this, enabling them to maintain 90 percent or superior performance. CKD is most commonly identified by coincidence at this stage during normal blood and urine testing. These tests may also be performed if you have diabetes or high blood pressure, which are the leading causes of CKD in the United States.

**SYMPTOMS**

When the kidneys work at 90% or above, there are usually no symptoms.

**TREATMENT**

You may decrease illness development by doing the following:

1. If you have diabetes, work on controlling your blood sugar levels.

2. If you have hypertension, follow your doctor's recommendations for decreasing your blood pressure.

3. Maintain a well-balanced diet.

4. Tobacco should not be used.

5. Engage in physical exercise for at least 30 minutes each day, 5 days per week.

6. Maintain a weight that is acceptable for your body. If you don't currently visit a kidney specialist (nephrologist), get a referral from your primary care physician.

**STAGE 2**

Slight reductions in renal function 60-89 mL/min 60-89%.

Kidneys in stage 2 function between 60 and 89 percent of the time.

## SYMPTOMS

You may still be symptom-free at this point. Or the symptoms are general, such as ;
1. Fatigue.
2. Itching.
3. Appetite loss.
4. Sleep issues.
5. Weakness

## TREATMENT

It's time to start working with a renal expert. Although there is no cure for CKD, early therapy may halt or stop its development. It is critical to treat the underlying cause. If you have diabetes, high blood pressure, or heart disease, follow your doctor's recommendations for treatment. Maintaining a healthy diet, getting regular exercise, and controlling your weight is also crucial. Ask your doctor about smoking cessation programs if you smoke.

**STAGE 3**

A mild-to-moderate reduction in renal function 45-59 mL/min 45-59%

Kidney illness in its third stage Stage 3A kidney function ranges between 45 and 59 percent. Kidney function is between 30 and 44 percent in stage 3B. The kidneys are not filtering waste, poisons, and fluids effectively, and they are beginning to accumulate.

**SYMPTOMS**

Stage 3 symptoms do not affect everyone. However, you may have;

1. Backache.

2. Weariness appetite loss.

3. Sleep issues due to constant itching Hand and foot swelling.

4. Urinating more or less than normal.

5. Weakness.


**COMPLICATIONS**

Possible complications include:

1. Bone disease.

2. Anemia.

3. Blood pressure that is too high.

**TREATMENT**

To help protect kidney function, it is critical to address underlying diseases. This might include:
1. High blood pressure drugs, such as angiotensin-converting enzyme (ACE) inhibitors or angiotensin II receptor blockers, diuretics.

2. A reduced salt diet to decrease fluid retention, and cholesterol-lowering medications.

3. Anemia erythropoietin supplements.
Phosphate binders to avoid calcification in blood vessels after a decreased protein diet so your kidneys don't have to work as hard

4. Vitamin D supplements to treat deteriorating bones You'll most likely need regular follow-up visits and testing so that modifications may be made as needed. Your doctor might send you to a dietician to ensure you are receiving enough nutrients.

**STAGE 4**

Kidney illness in the fourth stage You have moderate-to-severe renal damage if you are at stage 4. They're only working 15 to 29 percent of the time,(mild-to-moderate impairment of renal function 30-44 mL/min 30-44%).

so you might be accumulating extra waste, poisons, and fluids in your body. You must do all possible to avoid renal failure. According to the CDC, 48 percent of persons with significantly impaired kidney function are unaware of their condition.

## SYMPTOMS

Common symptoms include:

1. Backache.
2. Chest discomfort.
3. Diminished mental acuity.
4. Fatigue.
5. Appetite's loss.
6. Twitches or cramps in the muscles.
7. Vomiting and nausea.
8. Itching that doesn't go away.
9. Shortness of breath.
10. Sleep issues.

11. Hand and foot swelling weakness.

12. urinating more or less than normal Possible.

## COMPLICATIONS

Complications include:

1. Bone disease

2. Anemia

3. Blood pressure that is too high

4. You're also more likely to develop heart disease or have a stroke.

## TREATMENT

Treatment You'll need to collaborate closely with your physicians at stage 4. In addition to the same therapy as in previous phases, you should consider dialysis and kidney transplantation if your kidneys fail. These processes need precise organization and a lot of time, so it's best to start planning early.

## STAGE 5

Kidney illness at the fifth stage Stage 5 indicates that your kidneys are operating at less than 15%

capacity or that you have renal failure(Significant declines in renal function 15-29 mL/min 15-29% 5% renal failure 15 mL/min).

When this occurs, the accumulation of waste and pollutants becomes lethal. This is a case of end-stage renal disease.

**SYMPTOMS**
Kidney failure symptoms may include:
back and chest aches
breathing difficulties reduced mental acuity weariness little to no appetite muscular twitching or spasms constant stinging and nausea difficulty sleeping serious ailments Hand and foot swelling urinating more or less than normal Heart disease and stroke are becoming more common.

**TREATMENT**
Without dialysis or a kidney transplant, life expectancy after full renal failure is just a few months.

**DIALYSIS** is not a cure for kidney illness, but rather a method of removing waste and fluid from the circulation. Dialysis is classified into two types: hemodialysis and peritoneal dialysis.

*Hemodialysis* is performed in a dialysis facility regularly, generally three times each week. Two needles are inserted into your arm before each therapy. They are connected to a dialyzer, which is also known as an artificial kidney. The filter filters your blood and returns it to your body. Although you may be taught to do this at home, creating venous access needs a surgical procedure.

Home dialysis is more common than treatment center dialysis.

*Peritoneal Dialysis*: Dialysis via the peritoneum A catheter will be surgically implanted into your belly for peritoneal dialysis. During treatment, dialysis solution goes via the catheter into the abdomen, and then you may resume your daily activities. After a few hours, empty the catheter into a bag and discard it. This must be done 4 to 6 times each day.

***Kidney Transplant***: includes the replacement of your damaged kidney with a healthy one. Kidneys may be obtained from either live or dead donors. You will not need dialysis, but you will be required to take anti-rejection medicines.

# CHAPTER 3: CAUSES OF CHRONIC KIDNEY DISEASE

The most prevalent causes of chronic kidney disease (CKD) are diabetes and high blood pressure. Your doctor will examine your medical history and may order tests to determine the cause of your kidney illness. The sort of therapy you get may be affected by the etiology of your kidney illness.

*1. Diabetes*: Too much glucose, often known as sugar, in your blood harms the filters in your kidneys. Your kidneys might become so damaged over time that they no longer filter wastes and excess fluid from your blood. Protein in the urine is often the first indicator of kidney damage caused by diabetes. When the filters are destroyed, a protein called albumin, which is essential for your health, leaks from your blood into your urine. A healthy kidney prevents albumin from passing from the blood into the urine. Diabetic renal disease is the medical name for diabetes-related kidney disease.

**2. _Blood pressure:_** that is too high High blood pressure may damage blood vessels in the kidneys, causing them to perform less efficiently. If the blood arteries in your kidneys are damaged, your kidneys may be unable to eliminate wastes and excess fluid from your body as effectively. Extra fluid in the blood arteries may cause blood pressure to rise even higher, creating a deadly cycle.

Other reasons for kidney disease Other causes of kidney disease include as follows:

**3. _Polycystic kidney disease_** (PKD) is a hereditary illness that causes numerous cysts to form in the kidneys. an infection a medicine that is harmful to the kidneys an illness that affects the whole body, such as diabetes or lupus NIH external link.

**4. _Lupus nephritis_** is the medical term for kidney illness caused by lupus IgA glomerulonephritis. Anti-GBM (Goodpasture's) disease heavy metal poisoning, such as lead poisoning NIH external link Alport syndrome, for example, is a rare hereditary disorder NIH external link IgA vasculitis renal artery stenosis hemolytic uremic syndrome in children

# CHAPTER 4 : HOW TO MANAGE KIDNEY DISEASE

1. Maintain a healthy blood pressure level. If you have diabetes, meet your blood glucose target. Controlling your blood pressure is the most critical action you can do to address renal disease. High blood pressure may cause kidney injury. You can preserve your kidneys by maintaining your blood pressure at or below the level recommended by your doctor. Blood pressure should be less than 140/90 mm Hg for the majority of individuals. Develop a strategy with your healthcare provider to reach your blood pressure targets.

Steps you may take to accomplish your blood pressure objectives include eating heart-healthy, low-sodium meals, stopping smoking, getting enough exercise, getting enough sleep, and taking your medications as directed.

Check your blood glucose level frequently to achieve your blood glucose target. Use the findings to make choices regarding diet, exercise, and medications. Inquire with your doctor about how often you should monitor your blood glucose level.

Your A1C will also be tested by your doctor. The A1C test is a blood test that determines your average blood glucose level over the last three months. This test is distinct from the routine blood glucose tests you do.

The higher your A1C score, the higher your blood glucose levels during the last three months. Maintain a careful eye on your daily blood glucose levels to help you reach your A1C target.

Many patients with diabetes have an A1C target of less than 7%. Inquire with your doctor about your desired outcome. Reaching your target levels will assist you in protecting your kidneys. Learn more about diabetes management.

2. Monitor your kidney health with the help of your medical team. Take medications exactly as directed. The tests used by doctors to diagnose kidney illness may also be used to monitor changes in kidney function and damage. Kidney disease deteriorates with time. Ask your provider how the test findings compare to the previous ones every time you are examined. Your objectives will be to maintain your GFR constant and Maintain or reduce your urine albumin levels.

3. Create a food plan with the help of a dietician.

4. Include physical exercise in your daily routine.

5. Strive towards a healthy weight.

6. Get adequate rest.

7. Quit smoking.

8. Discover healthy coping mechanisms for stress and despair.

9. Maintain a healthy blood pressure level.

## HOW CAN I PREPARE FOR MY DOCTOR'S APPOINTMENTS?

The more you prepare ahead of time for your appointments, the more you will learn about your health and treatment choices. Make a list of inquiries. It's natural to have many questions. Write down your questions as you think of them so you remember everything you want to ask your healthcare provider when you visit him or her.

You may want to inquire about the tests being performed, the meaning of the findings, or the modifications you must make to your diet and medications. Sample questions to ask your doctor if you have kidney illness Concerning your testing What is the value of my GFR? What does this imply? Has my GFR altered since the last time I checked? What is the albumin level in my urine? What does it imply? Is my urine albumin level different from the previous time it was checked? Is my renal illness worsening? Is my blood pressure in the normal range? Concerning treatment and self-care What can I do to protect my sickness from worsening?

Do any of my medications or dosages need to be adjusted? When should I take each of my medications? Do I need to adjust my diet? Will you recommend a nutritionist for dietary advice? When will I need the services of a nephrologist (a kidney specialist)?

Is it necessary for me to consider dialysis or a kidney transplant? What should I do to protect my veins? Concerning complications What additional health issues can I encounter as a result of my kidney disease? Should I be on the lookout for any symptoms? If so, what exactly are they? Bring a friend or family for moral support. A trusted friend or family member may assist you recall what the provider said during the visit by taking notes, asking questions you may not have thought of, offering support, and taking notes. Discuss your expectations for the visit and the role you want your friend or family to perform ahead of time.

## WHO MAKES UP MY MEDICAL TEAM?

The following health care professionals may be engaged in your treatment as part of the health care team:

*1. Primary Care Physician.* The person you see for regular medical appointments is your primary care provider (PCP), who might be a doctor, nurse practitioner, or physician assistant. Your primary care physician may monitor your kidney function and assist you in managing diabetes and high blood pressure.

A primary care physician may also prescribe medications and refer you to specialists. Nurse.

*2. A nurse* may assist you with your therapy and educate you about kidney disease monitoring and treatment, as well as managing your health concerns. Some nurses focus on renal illness.

**3. *A dietitian who is registered*.** A certified dietician is a food and nutrition specialist who assists persons with renal disease in developing a healthy eating plan. Dietitians may assist you by developing an eating plan depending on the state of your kidneys.

**4. *Renal dietitians*** are typically found at dialysis facilities and are specifically trained to help clients who have renal failure. Diabetes instructor.

**5. *A diabetes educator,*** educates diabetics on how to control their condition and deal with diabetes-related issues.

**6. *Pharmacist.*** A pharmacist helps you understand your medications and fills your prescriptions. The pharmacist's work includes reviewing all of your medications, including over-the-counter (OTC) medications and supplements, to prevent dangerous combinations and adverse effects.

**7. *Worker in social services.*** When you are on the verge of requiring dialysis, you may be able to visit with a social worker. A dialysis social worker assists persons and their families in coping with the life changes and expenses associated with kidney disease and kidney failure. A dialysis social worker may also assist persons with renal failure in applying for financial assistance to meet treatment expenses.

**8. *Nephrologist.*** A nephrologist is a doctor who specializes in kidney disease. If you have a difficult case of kidney disease, your renal illness is rapidly worsening, or your kidney disease is advanced, your PCP may send you to a nephrologist.

## MANAGEMENT

1. Take medications exactly as directed. Many persons with CKD use medications to regulate their blood pressure, blood glucose, and

cholesterol. You may also need to take a diuretic, sometimes known as a water pill. The objective is to achieve your blood pressure target. If you decrease your salt consumption, these medications may function better.

2. Understand that your medications may alter over time. As your kidney condition worsens, your doctor may adjust your medications. Your kidneys aren't filtering as efficiently as they used to, which might lead to a hazardous accumulation of medications in your blood. Some medications might potentially be harmful to your kidneys. As a consequence, your service provider may advise you to take medication less often or at a lower dosage.

3. Stop using a medication or switch to another one Your pharmacist and health care provider should be aware of any medications you are taking, including OTC medications, vitamins, and supplements. Discuss with your physician all of the medications you use, including OTC medications, vitamins, and supplements.

4. Take caution while using over-the-counter medications. You may be using nonsteroidal anti-inflammatory drugs (NSAIDs) if you use over-the-counter or prescription medications for headaches, discomfort, fever, or colds. NSAIDs are regularly used pain relievers and cold medications that might harm your kidneys and cause acute renal injury, particularly in those who have kidney disease, diabetes, or high blood pressure.

NSAIDs include ibuprofen and naproxen. Because NSAIDs are offered under a variety of brand names, ask your pharmacist or healthcare provider whether the medications you are taking are safe to use. NSAIDs may also be seen on Drug Facts labels, such as the one below:
A nonsteroidal anti-inflammatory medicine (NSAID) medicine Facts label displaying the active component ibuprofen and its use as a pain treatment. If you've been using NSAIDs daily to relieve chronic pain, you should talk to your doctor about alternative options, such as meditation or other relaxation methods.

# CHAPTER 5: WAYS TO HELP YOUR FRIEND OR FAMILY MEMBER WITH KIDNEY FAILURE

Seeing someone you care about suffer from renal failure may be terrifying and distressing. You may feel befuddled and unaware of how to assist.

Here are five ways you may help a loved one who is suffering from renal failure.

*1. Learn About Their Treatment Strategy.* When your kidneys are healthy, they eliminate wastes and excess fluid from your blood; however, when your kidneys fail, toxins may build up in your blood and make you unwell. Dialysis helps the kidneys by removing toxins and fluid, allowing individuals with end-stage renal disease to feel better and live longer lives.

Knowing what kind of dialysis your loved one is on will help you better comprehend their situation and assist them properly.

People with renal failure may need to reduce their salt, phosphorus, potassium, and fluid consumption in addition to dialysis treatments. Protein may be lost during the dialysis procedure, thus they may need to consume additional high-protein meals.

*2. Pool Resources:* Unless you've experienced renal failure, you're unlikely to fully get what your friend or family member is going through or have all the solutions. That's fine! What you can do is provide them with materials to help them on their path where you cannot.

*3. Assist them in locating a live donor:* A kidney transplant may enhance the quality of life for many individuals, but there aren't enough kidneys to go around. While the NKF works tirelessly to guarantee that kidney transplants are accessible to everyone in need, there are currently over 100,000 individuals on the waiting list and not enough donors to go around. But don't give up hope. People from many walks of life are pitching in to make others' lives better, including family, friends, and strangers.

Sharing openly who you are, who loves you, and how tough it is to live with kidney failure might help prospective donors connect with your narrative. Even if they are not inclined to donate, they may feel compelled to share the tale and help spread the news.

4. Be precise Instead of a general "let me know how I can help," provide particular tasks that you are comfortable completing. This may be advantageous, particularly for people who have difficulties accepting aid.

Here are a few suggestions to get you started:
*Attend their dialysis appointment. Bring over
*kidney-friendly dishes.
*Offer to babysit children or pets.
*Help around the home or in the yard Listen

**5. *Keep an eye out for signs of sadness.*** Kidney failure may make a person feel ill and is often accompanied by worry, tension, and disorientation. With all of the changes, it's hardly surprising that they'd suffer despair.

However, since certain symptoms of depression and renal failure are similar, many persons on dialysis may be unaware that they have depression

These are some examples:

*Fatigue

*Sleep issues

*Appetite problems

*Headaches

*Irritability comes from a lack of attention.

*Swings in the mood.

Other symptoms of depression include a loss of interest in typical activities, recurrent angry outbursts, drug addiction, and social isolation. If you see these changes, encourage them to express their emotions and seek expert assistance. Their renal doctor, nurse, or social worker can help them evaluate whether they have depression and which treatment choice is best for them.

Conclusion

If you have anyone having kidney disease treat them with care,as what they need is your care, attention and understanding. At this point of their lives they need someone who could understand both their emotions too.

Encourage them and pray with them.